Health Benefits of Almonds

I0420694

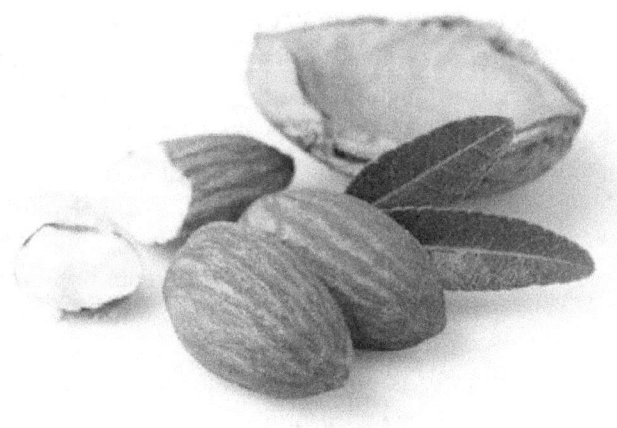

By M.Usman

Health Learning Series

Mendon Cottage Books

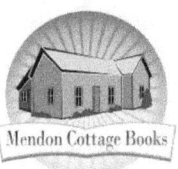

JD-Biz Publishing

Download Free Books!

http://MendonCottageBooks.com

Disclaimer

The information is this book is provided for informational purposes only. It is not intended to be used and medical advice or a substitute for proper medical treatment by a qualified health care provider. The information is believed to be accurate as presented based on research by the author.

The contents have not been evaluated by the U.S. Food and Drug Administration or any other Government or Health Organization and the contents in this book are not to be used to treat cure or prevent disease or mental illness.

The author or publisher is not responsible for the use or safety of any diet, procedure or treatment mentioned in this book. The author or publisher is not responsible for errors or omissions that may exist.

Warning

The Book is for informational purposes only and before taking on any diet, treatment or medical procedure it is recommended to consult with your primary care provider.

Check out some of the other Health Learning Series books at Amazon.com

Health Learning Series on Amazon

Download Free Books!
http://MendonCottageBooks.com

Table of Contents

Getting Started

Chapter # 1: Intro

Uniquely delicious, almonds have been known to man as the epitome of health & wellbeing for centuries. Their health benefits have been documented with the passage of time and are now being tested in the light of modern scientific researches; looking at the results of these researches, there is a good reason why you should consider reading the rest of the book!

A stalwart nut in cakes, puddings and other sweat dishes, almonds have been on almost every household's shopping list. With respect to freshness, they are always preferred to hazelnuts & walnuts and their slow rate of rancidity makes them a food item that can easily tolerate the back of a storage cupboard. Their neutral, nutty and crunchy taste upon baking makes them irresistibly delicious and in no time can you nibble your way through every almond in front of you.

But what are the origins of this super-delicious and nutritious food? Almond is actually a species of trees, belonging to the genus Prunus, which are indigenous to the South & Middle East region of Asia. The almond plant is widely cultivated for its edible seed, also known as almond. The almond tree is a deciduous one and grows 4-10 m in height; it has a trunk of diameter 30 cm. The twigs when young are of green color but become purplish as soon as they are exposed to sunlight. In the second year the twigs become grey and the leaves grow 3-5 inches long. The flowers are characterized by white to pinkish color, 3-5 cm diameter and usually consist of 5 petals. The fruit matures in the autumn, about 8 months after flowering but still for an economic bearing, one more year is required. The fruit is about 4-6 cm long and in specific terms is not exactly a nut, but rather a drupe. A drupe is a fruit in which an outer fleshy part surrounds a shell containing a seed but instead of being fleshy the outer part of the fruit is thick and leathery in texture. Inside this hull is a hard, woody shell which packs the edible seed known to many as almond. The seed acquired from the woody shell is covered by a thin brownish skin, which when pealed reveals the inner color of almond; i.e. off white. Almonds can further be categorized into two types:

i.   Sweet Almonds

ii.   Bitter Almonds

Sweet almonds are the ones that are generally consumed; oval in shape, they are usually malleable in texture & soothingly buttery in taste. In the market, shelled almonds can be found in whole, slivered or sliced form; in either their natural form or with their skin removed.

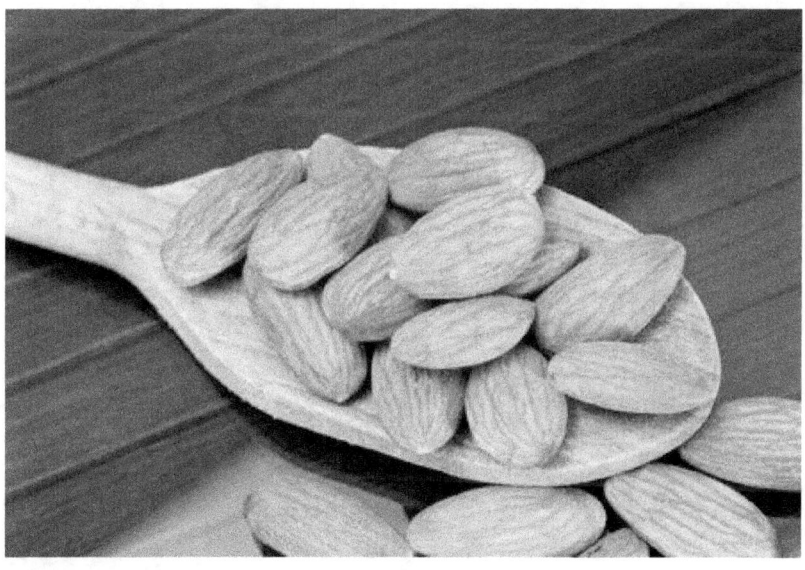

Bitter almonds on the other hand are made into almond oil that is used as a flavoring agent in foods and liqueurs. Otherwise, as the name suggests, they are inedible and contain toxic compounds like hydrocyanic acid. (These compounds are removed while processing to produce almond oil)

The almond is native to the Middle Eastern region of Asia, which has a similar climate to the Mediterranean. It was spread into Northern Africa and Southern Europe by travelers in ancient times, most recent of which was the spreading of almonds to parts of the new world, i.e. California. There is also a wild form of almonds that grows in the Levant, which is transformed into poison by crushing, chewing or inflicting any other injury to the seed. It still remains a mystery as to how humans chose sweet almonds and cultivated them.

Almonds are loaded with minerals, vitamins, fiber and proteins which are associated with several nurturing health benefits for the body; just a handful of almonds (1 ounce) can fill up to $1/8^{th}$ of your body's protein tank! The nuts are also a well-supplied source of energy other than being loaded with nutrients. They are highlighted for their richness in mono-unsaturated fatty acids that help to lower bad cholesterol and at the same time raise levels of good cholesterol in the body. A great amount of vitamin E can also be acquired from almonds (1/4 of almonds is vitamin E) which is a very powerful antioxidant required by the body for the maintenance of cell membranes and protecting cells against free radical oxygen damage.

Almond is gluten free and can therefore be enjoyed by people of all sorts, gluten intolerant or not; it can be a healthy alternative for those with the celiac disease. Almond oil is another useful by product of almonds and can be used to tackle a variety of skin problems. All in all, by munching away on almonds you can help not only ward of life threatening diseases but also help your body accomplish many of the tasks that require a good & constant supply of minerals and nutrients.

If words are still not enough, you should let the numbers do the talking; the world produced an astonishing 2 million tons of almonds in the year 2011, alone. The US was the largest producer of almonds followed by countries in the Mediterranean and Middle East. This wonder of nature is moreover available round the year, which makes it all the more attractive to nut lovers & enthusiasts.

Keep on reading and soon you'll discover why you should have started consuming this gift from nature a long time ago and why it's still not too late.

Chapter # 2: Nutritional Worth

An ounce of almonds that are more or less 25 in number contain about 12% of our daily protein requirements. They are a rich source of vitamin B, E and essential minerals like calcium, potassium and magnesium. Last but not the least, they also contain phytosterols which are compounds associated with lowering cholesterol.

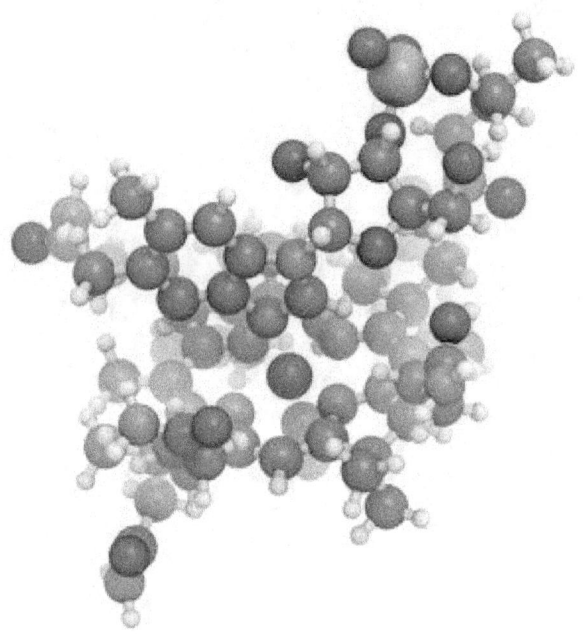

Almonds are a great source of alpha-tocopherol, the type of vitamin E that is most easily absorbed by the body. Vitamin E works as an antioxidant in the body; it helps muscles by preventing post-workout free-radical damage that result in muscle strain and cell destruction. The less free radical damage there is, the faster the muscles can recover and more you can benefit from the workout. Vitamin E is also noted for preventing cognitive decline, preserving memory longer, boosting alertness and protecting against UV rays. B vitamins are another type of essential combination of vitamin which is mainly essential for energy production in the body. If the right amount of B vitamins is consumed on a daily basis, the body can benefit from it in the form of increased athletic performance, strength and healthy body parts. Almonds also contain "healthy fats" or monounsaturated fats that help to decrease bad or LDL cholesterol from the bloodstream, reducing the risk of heart diseases.

Almonds are also a combined source of calcium, potassium and magnesium which are all undoubtedly very useful nutrients; but these minerals gain their real power when they are combined and that's when they really benefit the body. One such combination is vitamin E, potassium, magnesium and calcium; these minerals together are very essential for the production of testosterone which is very useful for men over 30 who feel decline in this hormone. Another such combo is vitamin E, B and magnesium, which work together to improve the immunity system of the body.

A detailed account of the nutritional wellness of almonds is given in the following table. The amount per 1 cup taken is 95 grams.

Calorie Information	
Nutrient	**Amount**
Total Calories	546
From Carbohydrates	83.3
From Fat	393

From Proteins	70

Carbohydrates

Nutrient	Amount
Total Carbohydrates	20.6 g
Dietary Fiber	11.6 g
Starch	0.7 g
Sugar	3.7 g

Fats & Fatty Acids

Nutrient	Amount
Total Fat	47.0 g
Saturated Fat	3.5 g
Mono-saturated Fat	29.3 g
Polyunsaturated Fat	11.5 g
Total Omega-3 Fatty acids	5.7 mg
Total Omega-6 Fatty acids	11462 mg

Proteins

Nutrient	Amount
Protein	20.2 g

Vitamins

Nutrient	Amount
Vitamin E	24.9 mg
Thiamin	0.2 mg
Riboflavin	1.0 mg
Niacin	3.2 mg
Vitamin B6	0.1 mg
Folate	47.5 mcg

Vitamin B12	0.0 mg
Pantothenic Acid	0.4 mg
Choline	49.5 mg
Betaine	0.5 mg

Minerals

Nutrient	Amount
Calcium	251 mg
Iron	3.5 mg
Magnesium	255 mg
Phosphorus	460 mg
Potassium	670 mg
Sodium	1.0 mg
Zinc	2.9 mg
Copper	0.9 mg
Manganese	2.2 mg
Selenium	2.4 mcg

Chapter # 3: Selection & Storage

Almonds are nuts that are available in markets round the year. One can find different variants of almonds in a variety of stores such as shelled, unshelled, roasted, salted, powdered or sweetened. Almonds in their shell have the longest shelf life and therefore, should be your first preference if longevity is what you're looking for. If purchasing these, first shake the shells and if it rattles a lot the almond is most probably shrinking due to aging so leave it. Then check to see that the shells are not split, strained or moldy. If shelled almonds are being chosen, they should be packed in a hermetically sealed container since they will last longer than those sold in bulk bins which are exposed to all kinds of weather conditions like heat, humidity and air. With bulk bins, make sure that the bulk container remains sealed for most of the time when not in use and the store has a high turnover rate as this will ensure maximum freshness. In addition the smell of the almonds should be nutty but if the odor is sharp and bitter, the almonds have gone rancid. Also the chosen shelled nuts should be bright brown in color and have a solid feel to them. A quite easy rancidity check for shelled almonds, is slicing the almond in half and looking for a yellowish patch on the inner white surface; in case it turns out to be yellow the almond has gone way past its prime and should be thrown away immediately. When choosing unshelled almonds, make sure that the shells look uniform in color, not limping or shriveled.

On a similar note, if you need almonds with a roasted flavor & texture, choose the ones that have been "dry roasted" as they have not been cooked in any kind of oil unlike their counterparts. Even after making sure that dry roasted almonds are purchased, read the label to make sure that no additional ingredient like corn syrup, sugar or preservative of any kind has been added.

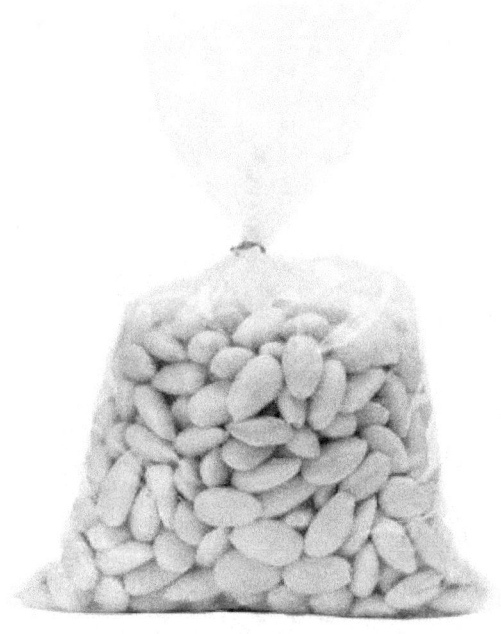

Coming to storage, since almonds have a high fat content (monounsaturated); it is therefore important that they are stored properly to prevent any rancidity from taking over. The first rule for storing almonds is that a hot pantry is rancidity's host. Shelled almonds should be stored in a tightly sealed container, in a cool, dark and dry place. Keeping them cold will further enhance their life time and ensure prolonged freshness for several months; if kept in a freezer, the lifetime can be extended to a whole year. According to the Almond Board of California, if unshelled almonds are kept in unopened packages in a cool, dark and dry environment, they can be stored for as long as two years.

Health Benefits

Chapter # 4: Lowering Cholesterol

Almonds are known to be high in fat and therefore, some people think that the idea of almonds lowering cholesterol is untrue. Well in reality, it's every bit as true; almonds are high in monounsaturated fats, the same type that are found in olive oil and are associated with the reducing risk of cardiovascular disease. Five very large human epidemiological studies were carried out to see any relation between almonds are risk of heart disease before moving onto detailed studies. The studies included Adventist health study, Nurses' health study, Physicians Health Study and Iowa Health Study all of which found that nut consumption was directly related to lowering the risk of heart disease. A rough estimate showed that substituting nuts with carbohydrates resulted in 30% reduction of the risk; the risk lowered further when saturated fats in the diet were replaced by fats from nuts.

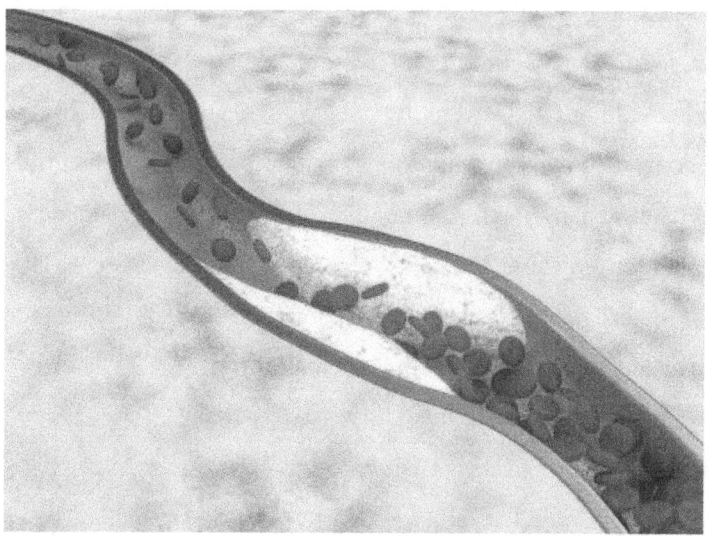

Another study published in the British Journal of Nutrition indicated that when foods that are known to lower LDL cholesterol are combined, their health promoting effects add together. In the study, 12 patients with elevated levels of LDL cholesterol were given a diet consisting of plant sterols, almonds, soy protein and soluble fiber (oats, pears and beans); the results showed that almost after 2 weeks, near maximal reductions were achieved, and that too of small dense LDL that is most notorious for increasing the risk of heart disease.

LDL is the cholesterol that is responsible for heart disease and atherosclerosis. In addition to the LDL lowering effects of almonds, the reduction of heart disease risk is also due to the antioxidant properties of vitamin E. The antioxidant characteristics of vitamin E prevent artery-clogging and free radical reactions in the body. A new study that was published in American Dietetic Association confirmed that consumption of almonds significantly raised the levels of vitamin E in the blood stream that helped reduce cholesterol. The research was conducted at Loma Linda University and it compared the effects of three different diets on healthy men and women for four weeks. The diets included a low-almond diet, a high-almond diet and a control diet that didn't include almonds at all. The low and high almond diets were prepared by replacing 10 and 20 percent of calories consumed daily with almonds; that amounts for 1-2 handfuls. It is to be noted that the participants did not take any multivitamin supplements throughout the study so the results were completely transparent. The results evaluated after 4 weeks showed that when people got 10% of their calories from almonds, the level of vitamin E increased by 13.7%. The effect was even greater for 20% and the level increased to 18.7%. Furthermore, the participants also lowered their LDL cholesterol by 7 percent.

Apart from vitamin E and monounsaturated fats, almonds also contain the minerals, magnesium and potassium. What is the importance of magnesium and potassium in the body? Magnesium can be considered as nature's pressure reliever; when there is enough magnesium in the body, the resistance on arteries and veins reduce and the flow of blood, nutrients and most importantly oxygen is improved. Studies have shown that those individuals suffering from a deficiency in magnesium not only have a higher risk of heart attack but also immediately after a heart attack is more vulnerable to free radical injury. Potassium, on the other hand is an important electrolyte, necessary for efficient nerve transmission and contraction of muscles in all parts of the body including the heart. A single cup of almonds provides the body with 670 mg of potassium, making them an exceptionally good choice for boosting up potassium supplies that ultimately help the heart against surges of high blood pressure.

Chapter # 5: Defense against Diabetes & Cardiovascular disease

Almonds can prove very effective in reducing the risk of diabetes by decreasing after meal rises in blood sugar and the free radicals damage that follows. Glycaemic index is a measure of the ability of a food to raise the level of glucose in blood sugar. Combining almonds with foods with high glycemic index reduces the food's index and therefore, lessens the rise in blood sugar.

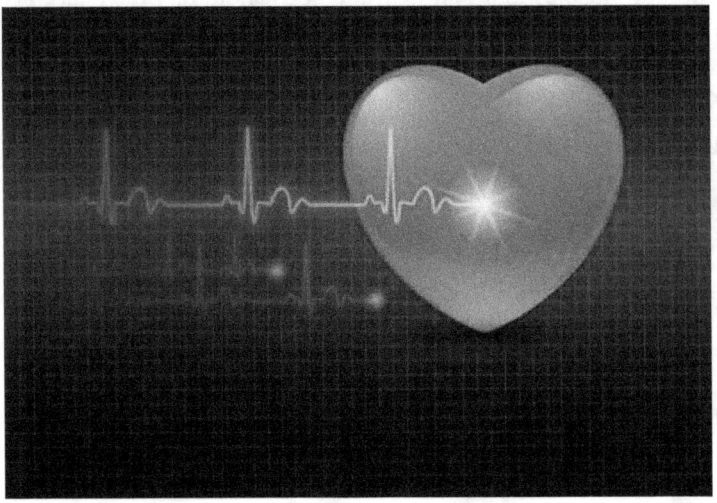

Fifteen healthy individuals were subjected to 5 meals providing different amounts of carbohydrates, proteins and fats. The test meals included almonds and bread, mashed potatoes and parboiled rice; there were also two bread control meals. When blood samples were taken before each meal and after 4 subsequent hours, the levels of protective antioxidants:

- Increased after the almond meal

- Decreased after every other meal

Other than increasing antioxidant levels, almond also lowered the rise in blood sugar after food had been consumed. In the study, an overnight 11 hours fast was observed by volunteers who were fed 3 test meals and 2 white breads meals on separate days. The meals contained 50 grams of carbohydrates each, from bread eaten either alone or in combination with 1-3 ounces of almonds. To ensure constant glucose pattern, blood samples were taken, immediately after eating and in 15 minutes intervals. It was found that almonds systematically reduced the glycemic index of the meal and rise in blood sugar. Furthermore, the amount of reduction was directly related to the amount of almonds consumed. When a single ounce of almonds was taken along with white bread the GI of the overall meal (105.8) was more or less equal to when bread was consumed alone, but when two almonds were consumed the GI dropped to 63; with three ounces the GI was only 45.2. Comparing the blood sugar levels, when the bread alone was consumed the blood sugar rose by 2.8 units.

- After an ounce of almonds were added to the bread, blood sugar rose by 2.2 units.

- After 2 ounces of almonds were added, the blood sugar rose by 2.0 units.

- After 3 ounces of almonds were added, the blood sugar rose by 1.6 units.

A way to include almonds in your diet is to buy almond butter and spread it on a toast or on the center of a stalk of celery. You can also add a handful of almonds that have been lightly roasted to your salad or chops or use it as a topping for steamed, sautéed vegetables and pasta.

Chapter # 6: Improves Blood Fats Levels

There is no need for people with a blood fat problem to shy away from high-fat snacks especially almonds. As described earlier, almonds contain monounsaturated fats that are good for the body. Researchers at the University of Toronto have successfully shown that 2.5 ounces of almonds every day can perform a better job at lowering LDL & raising HDL than a whole snack of wheat muffin that has the same amount of fiber and fats. It was also found that antioxidants in the body could be increased by compounds like phyto-nutrients, found in almonds and are believed to have special health promoting effects.

It is an established standard in the medical community that eating whole foods is the best way to combat illnesses and promote healthiness, and same is the case with almonds. Almonds should be consumed along with their skins as they contain flavonoids that bundle up with vitamin E found in the rest of the almond to deliver double the amount of antioxidants that are otherwise delivered. This study was published in the Journal of Nutrition where twenty potent antioxidant flavonoids were found to be residing in almond skins. Most of these were already recognized in the medical community for their benefits like *catechins* in green tea and naringenen in grapefruit. The team first tested the effects of flavonoids found in almond skin alone and then tested them in combination with vitamin E extracted from almond flesh. In case of flavonoids alone, the LDL's resistance to oxidation was enhanced by 18% but along with vitamin E, the LDL's resistance to oxidation was extended to 52.5%! This showed that whole foods were undoubtedly the best combination when it came to delivering a higher payload of the same benefit.

Chapter # 7: Weight Loss

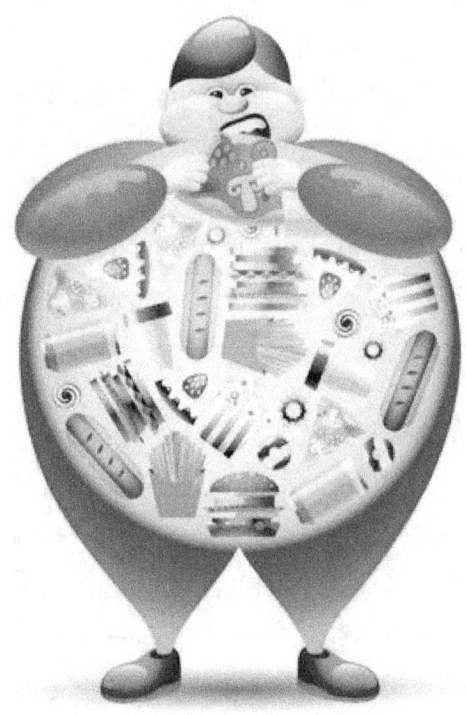

Obesity is one of the biggest chronic problems humanity is facing right now; people have become more and more indulged in artificial activities and prefer foods with high level of processing rather than healthy, natural ones. In this time of need almonds, which are already known for their nutritious properties have been discovered as a food item that works to help lose the body extra weight. A research was carried out on 65 overweight and obese adults with an almond-enriched calorie diet that concluded that the monounsaturated fats indeed helped the participants shed pounds more effectively when compared to a complex carbohydrate diet. The group that was on the almond-enriched diet consumed 39% of their share of calories from fat, 25% of which was categorized as monounsaturated. Those on the calorie diet that was high in complex carbohydrates consumed only 18% of their calories from fat (5% monounsaturated) whereas 53% of the calories were sourced from carbohydrates. Overall, both the diets supplied equal amounts of calories as well as proteins. After 6 months, those on the almond-enriched diet underwent greater reductions in weight, body fat, waistlines, body water and systolic blood pressure. The results can be stated as:

- 62% greater loss in BMI,
- 50% greater reduction in waist length and
- 56% more loss in body fat

On top of this, 96% of those participants who had type 1 diabetes reduced their medications to 50% compared to those on the high carb diet. The results were published in the International Journal of Obesity and Related Metabolic disorders.

Almonds not only help the body lose extra weight but they also prevent the weight from coming back. People who eat nuts like almonds at least twice a week are less likely to regain weight than those who never touch nuts. A 28 month study was carried out to prove this statement and involved 8,865 adult men & women from Spain. Participants who ate almonds and other nuts at least 2 times a week had 31% less chance of gaining weight than those who didn't ate nuts in that time period. Moreover, the participants who didn't eat nuts gained more weight in quantity than those who did. The conclusion by the authors stated that frequent nut consumption was successful in reducing risk of gaining 5kg or more weight hereby declaring that almond was undoubtedly diverse in its health promoting effects compared to other foods.

Chapter # 8: Normalizes Eating Habits

If you're still one of those who are reluctant to make almonds a part of their diet on grounds of high calorie count, a study in the British Journal of Nutrition might be the final nail in the coffin that would convince you to unlearn this myth. In the research, normal eating habits of 43 men and 38 women were studied for about 6 months. The participants were instructed to consume just about 2 ounces or a quarter cup of almonds on a daily basis along with no pressure to change any other part of their diet. At the end of the sixth month a number of changes were observed; the participants' intake of:

- Monounsaturated fatty acids increased by 42%.

- Polyunsaturated fatty acids increased by 24%.

- Fiber increased by 12%.

- Vegetable protein increased by 19%.

- Vitamin E increased by 66%.

- Copper increased by 15%.

- Magnesium increased by 23%.

While on the other hand, the intake of:

- Trans fatty acids decreased by 14%.

- Animal protein decreased by 9%.

- Sodium decreased by 21%.

- Cholesterol decreased by 17%.

- Sugars decreased by 13%.

The new set of changes closely resembled to the standards set out by health agencies showing that almond indeed helped in correcting faulty habits.

Apart from correcting eating habits, almonds can also help the body produce energy more efficiently by two of its very beneficial trace minerals, copper and manganese. Both of these are essential compounds for a key enzyme in the body called superoxide dismutase. This superoxide dismutase is responsible for disarming free radicals that are produced within the energy factories of our cells, the mitochondria. Presence of these trace minerals ensures a constant supply of energy throughout the body that is not under the load of the destructive free radicals.

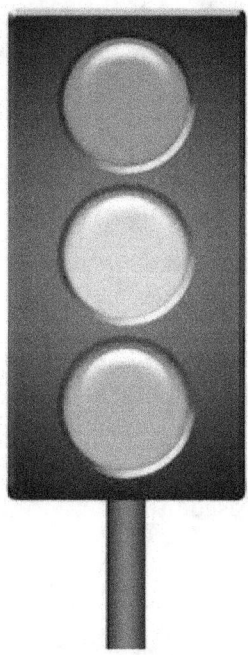

Vitamin B2 also plays important parts during the whole process of energy production. In the energy production pathways, vitamin B2 or riboflavin takes the form of FAD or FMN, both compounds that aid protein enzymes to allow oxygen-based energy production. These enzymes work throughout the body especially in areas of high oxygen-based energy production such as muscles and heart. Another benefit of riboflavin is defense of mitochondria from highly reactive oxygen free radicals. The body prevents damage from these free radicals by a molecule called glutathione, an antioxidant, but as with other hormones in the body, glutathione runs out and needs to be recycled. Vitamin B2 makes this recycling possible and indirectly prevents the mitochondria from any oxidizing damage.

Chapter # 9: Live Longer

Nature has provided cures to almost every disease but mortality is something not even technology can provide a fix to. At the maximum you can prolong your life for years to come but that's it; one such natural food that helps a person live longer is almond.

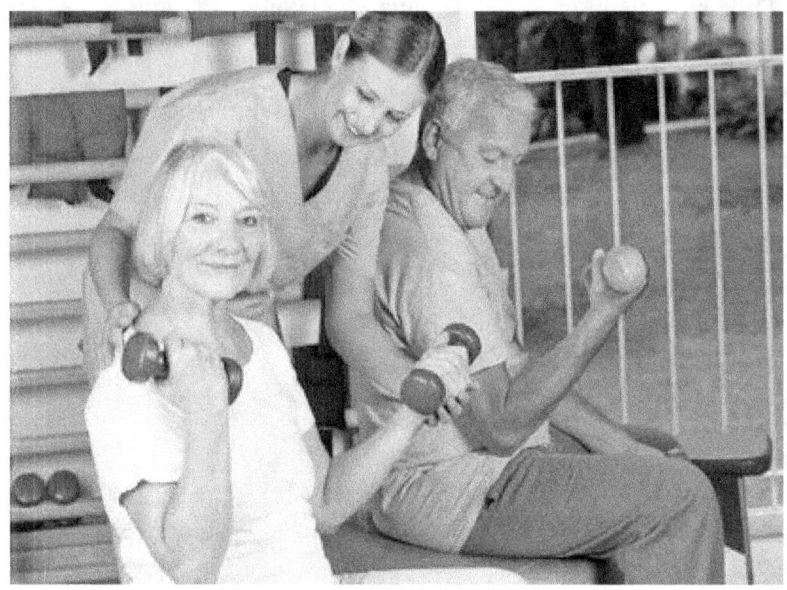

A very large study published in the New England Journal of Medicine showed that people who ate a handful of nuts every day lived longer than those who didn't. The study included scientists from Dana-Farber Cancer Institute & the Harvard School of Public Health who collected data of about 120,000 people over a span of 30 years. The analysis stated many of the revelations found out by smaller studies such as regular nut eaters tend to be slimmer than those who don't eat nuts, etc. The senior author of the study,

Professor Charles S. Fuchs said that the most obvious benefit of nuts was a 29% reduction in deaths from heart disease and 11% decrease from the risk of cancer. In the study, scientists first examined data from 1980 to 2010 collected from 76,464 women who took part in the Nurses' Health Study; 42,498 men soon followed whose data ranged from 1986 to 2010 and took part in the Health Professional's Follow-up Study. Each participant also filled detailed questionnaires every 2-4 years along with questions about their lifestyle and health in general. The questionnaire asked the participant to estimate the length of time before he/she had a 28g serving of nuts and to ensure fair results, the researchers used sophisticated statistical tools to rule out additional factors that may have a positive effect on the participant's health.

The results stated that consumption of nuts:

- Less than once a week was linked to 7% reduction in risk of death.

- Once a week, 11% reduction.

- 2-4 times a week, 13% reduction.

- 5-6 times a week, 15% reduction.

- Greater than 7 times a week, 20% reduction.

The results spoke for themselves and removed any doubt about the healthy and hearty characteristics of the wonder nut almond!

Chapter #10: Recipes

Candied Almonds

Makes: 2 cups

Prep time: 5 minutes

Cooking time: 15 minutes

Ready in: 35 minutes

Ingredients:

1. ½ cup water

2. 1 tablespoon ground cinnamon

3. 2 cups whole almonds

4. 1 cup white sugar

Directions:

Combine sugar, cinnamon and water in a saucepan and heat it over medium intensity until the mixture starts to boil. Add the almonds, stir the mixture until all the liquid has evaporated and syrup like coating is left on the almonds. Place the almonds in a baking sheet and separate them using a fork. Serve after cooling the almonds for a minimum of 15 minutes.

Sugar Spiced Almonds

Makes: 16 servings

Prep time: 5 minutes

Cooking time: 20 minutes

Ready in: 55 minutes

Ingredients:

1. 1 tablespoon olive oil

2. 1 tablespoon ground cinnamon

3. 1 pound blanched almonds

4. 3/8 teaspoon sweet paprika

5. ½ cup white sugar

6. ¼ teaspoon cayenne pepper

Directions:

Preheat your oven to 175 degrees Celsius. Combine olive oil and almonds in a bowl, spread them on a baking sheet and bake them in the oven until they are roasted, which takes about 15 minutes. While the almonds bake, mix cinnamon, paprika, sugar & cayenne pepper in a small bowl and sprinkle the mixture over almonds; bake the almonds once again until the spices are fragrant.

Garlic & Rosemary Roasted Almonds

Makes: 25 servings

Prep time: 10 minutes

Cooking time: 15 minutes

Ready in: 1hr 25 minutes

Ingredients:

1. 1 pound raw almonds

2. 4 sprigs fresh rosemary

3. 1 cup olive oil

4. ¼ teaspoon red pepper flakes

5. 4 cloves crushed garlic

6. Sea salt

Directions:

Preheat your oven to 175 degrees Celsius. Spread the almonds on a baking sheet and bake it in a preheated oven until the almonds turn golden brown & fragrant; this will take about 20 minutes. Transfer these hot almonds into a wide-bottomed glass. Heat garlic, olive oil, sea salt as per taste, rosemary leaves and red pepper flakes in a saucepan on low heat. In order to completely release the flavor, mash the garlic and rosemary in hot oil. Pour this hot oil mixture over the almonds that have been taken out and stir the new combination for 5-10 minutes until it completely cools. Finally, drain any oil from almonds and transfer them to a paper towel-lined plate.

Conclusion

Every research till now has shown that almond is a genuine health promoting wonder with benefits so diverse that they can't be found anywhere else, not in any other food item neither in any drug. Apart from curing ailments like heart disease and nerve damage, almonds can prolong a person's life time which for almost everyone is a killer feature! Everything about almond, from its types to its benefits to its recipes has been provided to you; the ball is in your court now and it's up to you to make a change out of it. All in all, almond is a top of the line, natural food item that can turn any person's life around and bring him back up to enjoy life and its pleasures.

Stay safe and enjoy!

References

http://nl.123rf.com/photo_15819737_gedroogde-van-amandelen.html

http://nl.123rf.com/photo_12083854_amandelen.html

http://nl.123rf.com/photo_18623668_gepelde-amandelen-geafa-soleerd-op-wit-in-zak-met-clipping-path.html

http://nl.123rf.com/photo_15968038_atherosclerose--medisch-concept.html

http://www.fotolia.com/id/39332640

http://www.fotolia.com/id/42606253

http://www.fotolia.com/id/49218655

http://www.fotolia.com/id/49728540

http://www.fotolia.com/id/58616701

Author Bio

Muhammad Usman is a distinguished medical graduate of Allama iqbal medical college (AIMC). He is a professional writer who has been in the field for more than 4 years. During this time he has produced 10,000+ articles, blogs and eBooks on various niches related to diseases, health, fitness, nutrition and well being. He is a regular contributor to several journals related to medicine and surgery. He is the editor of several journals and newspapers.

Check out some of the other Health Learning Series books at Amazon.com

Health Learning Series on Amazon

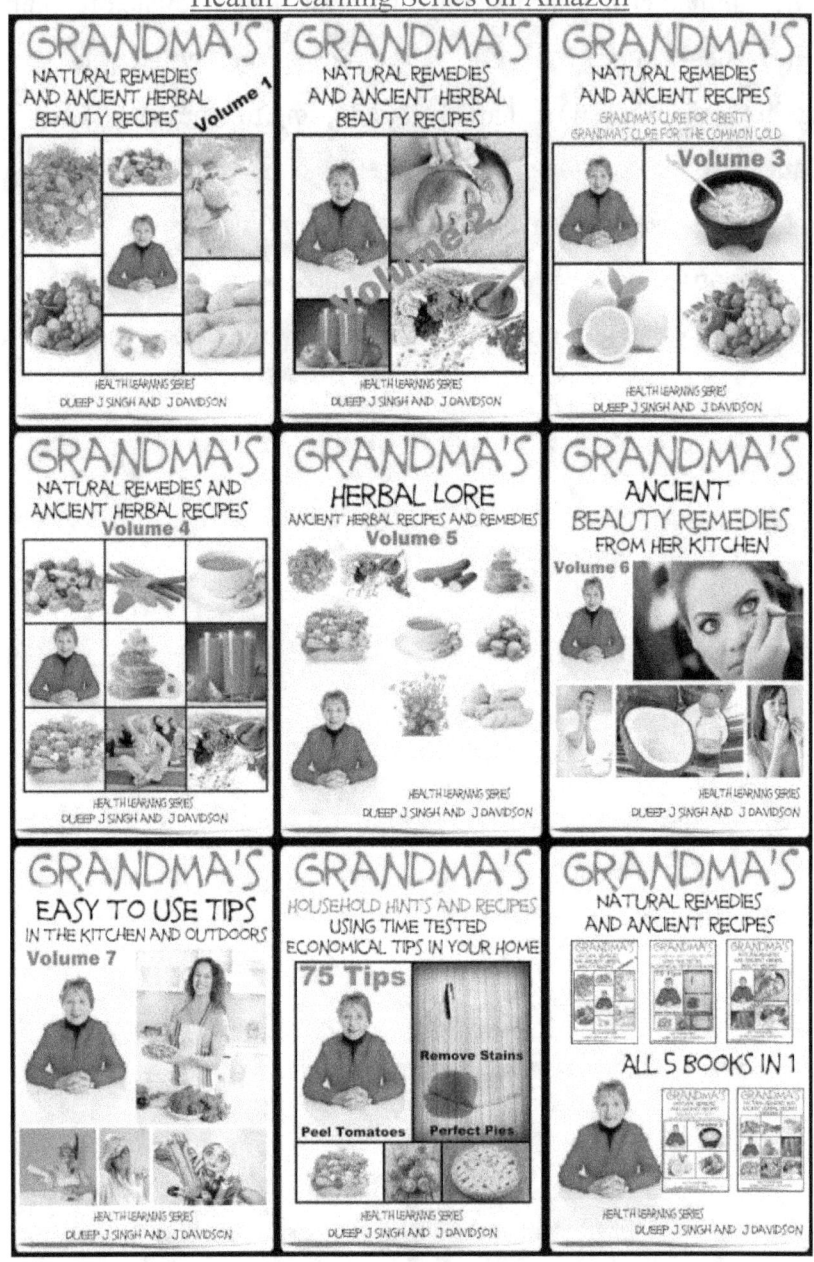

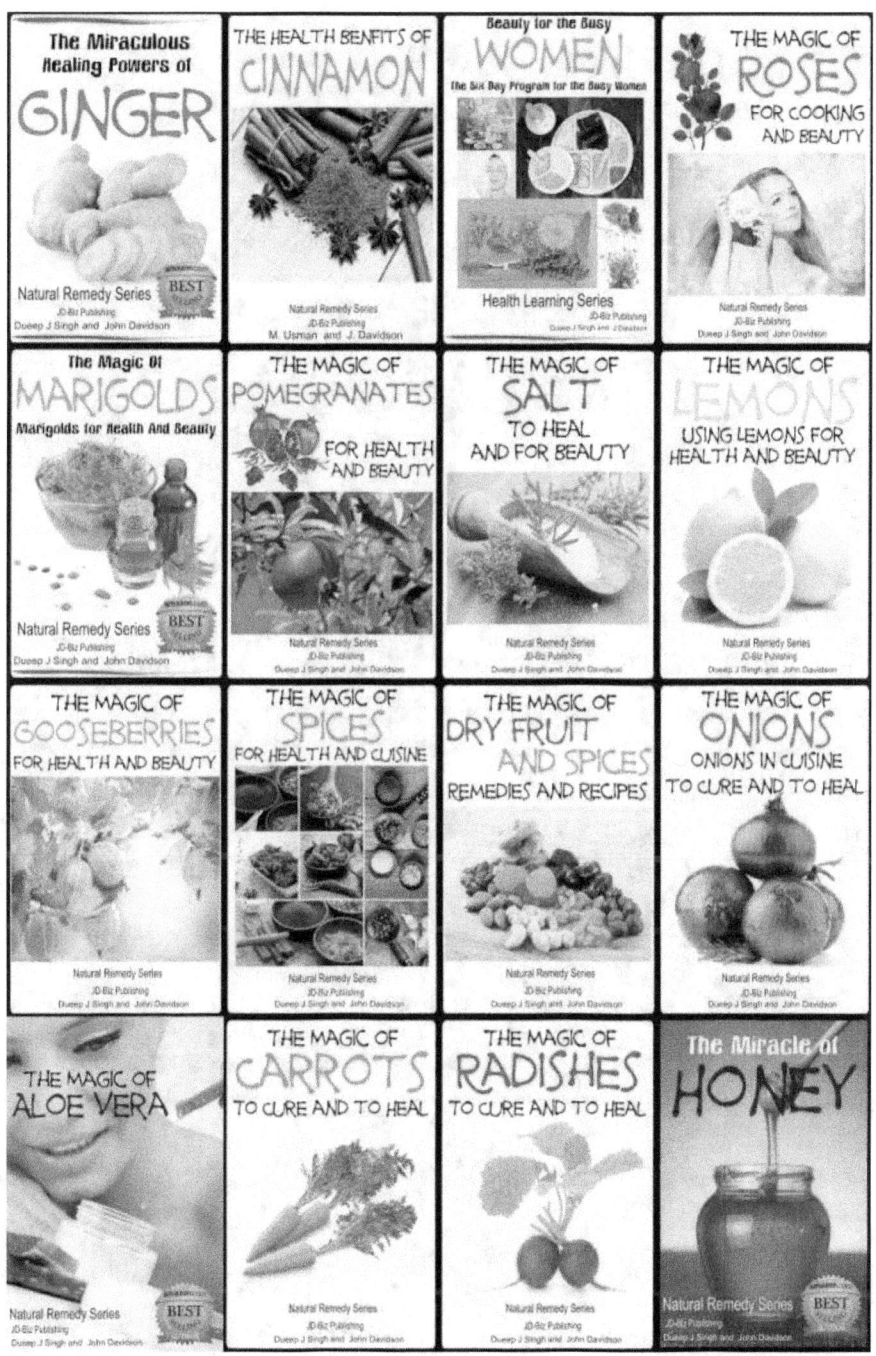

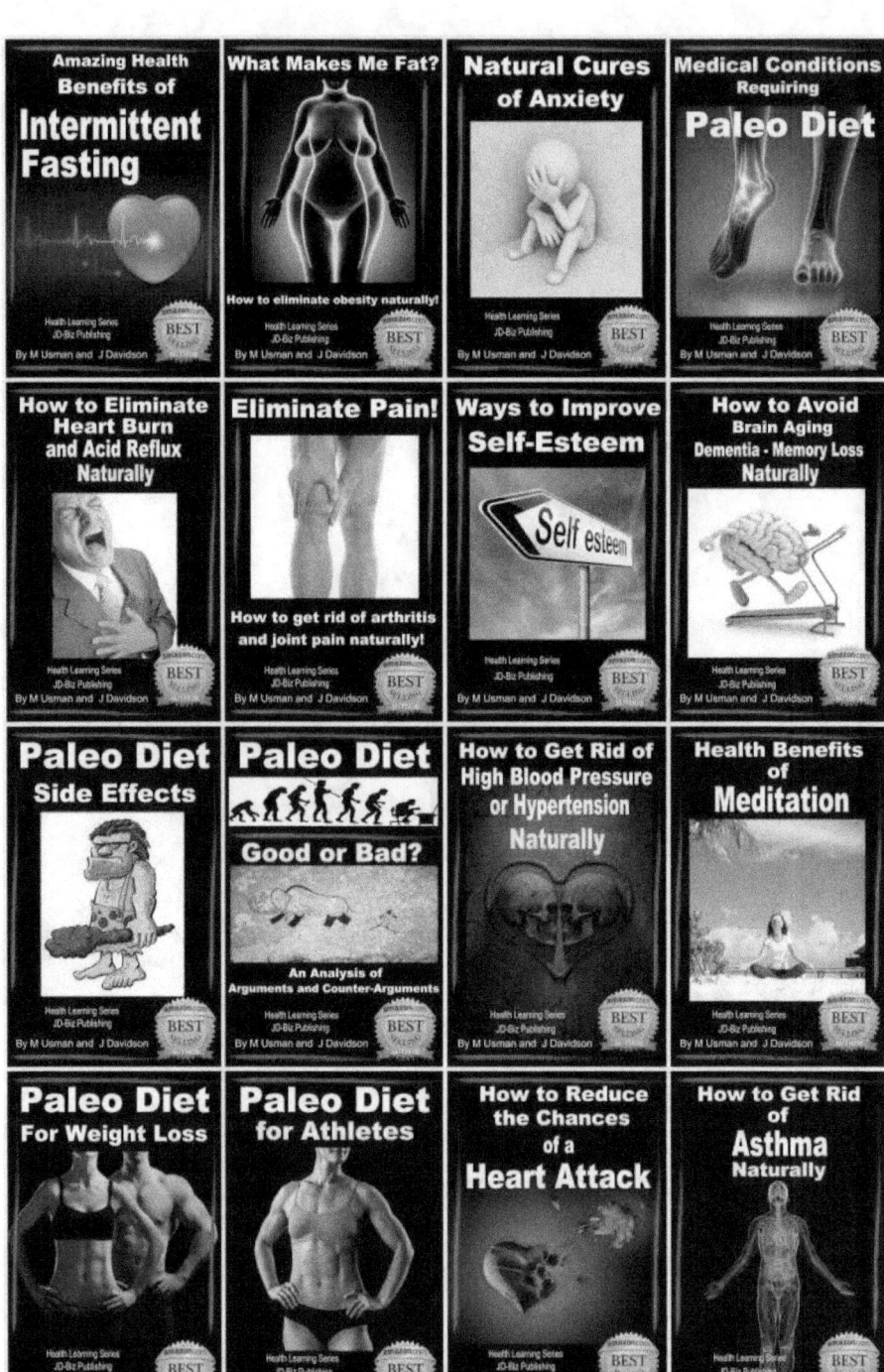

Amazing Animal Books Series

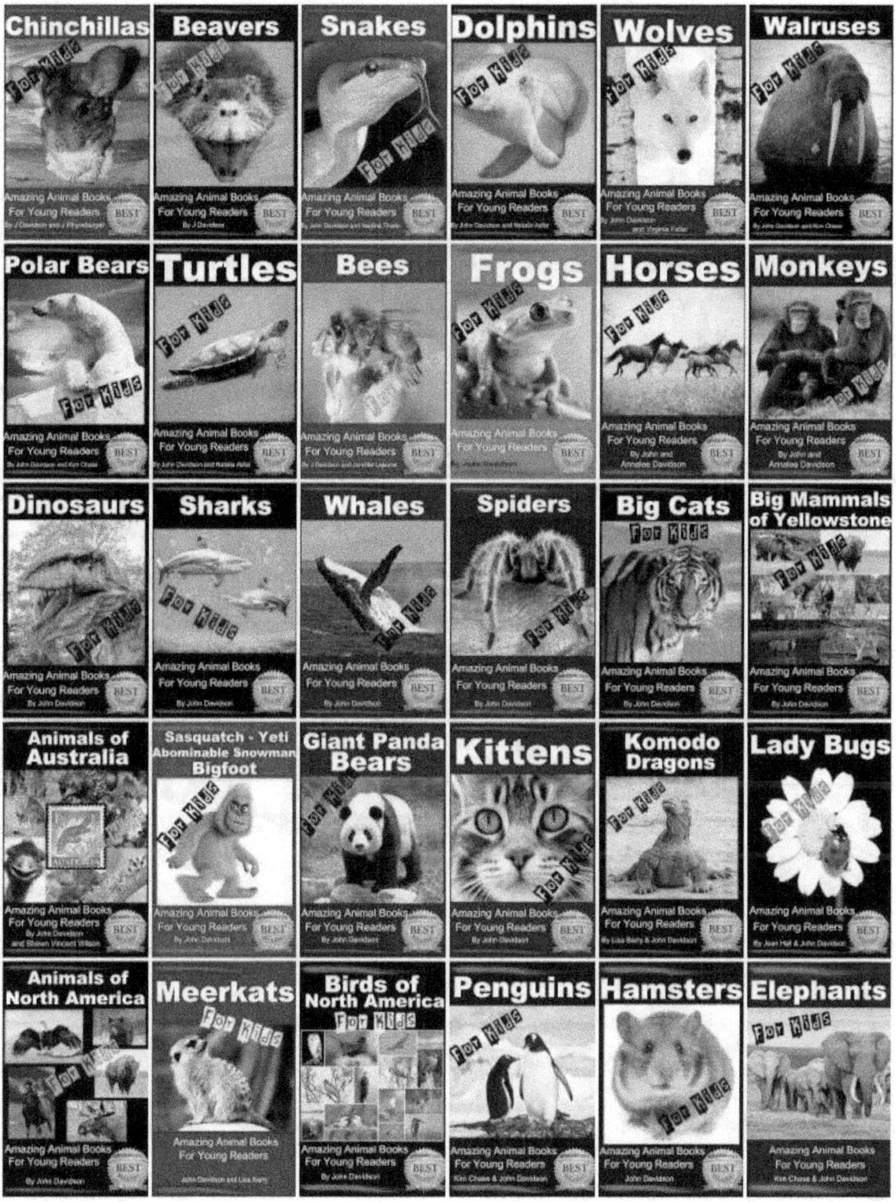

Learn To Draw Series

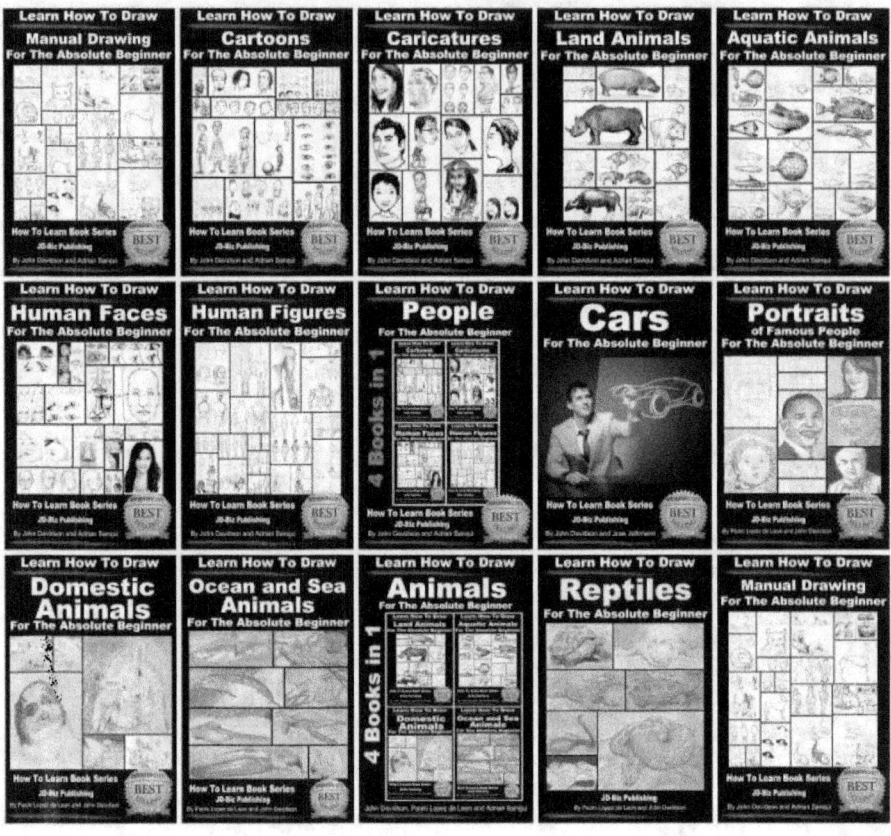

How to Build and Plan Books

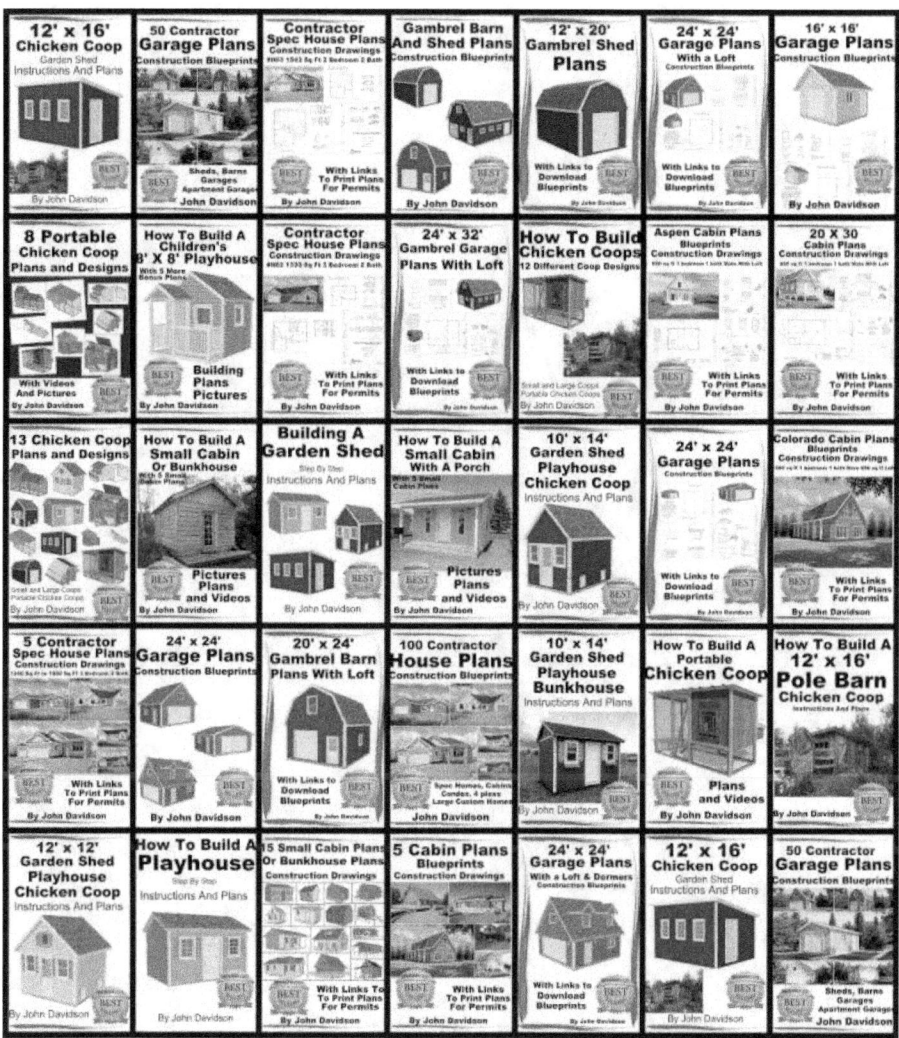

Our books are available at

1. Amazon.com

2. Barnes and Noble

3. Itunes

4. Kobo

5. Smashwords

6. Google Play Books

Download Free Books!

http://MendonCottageBooks.com

Publisher

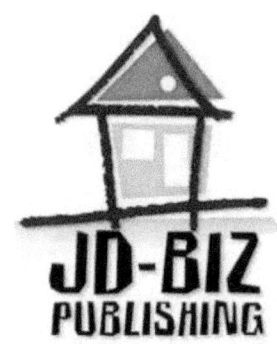

JD-Biz Corp

P O Box 374

Mendon, Utah 84325

http://www.jd-biz.com/

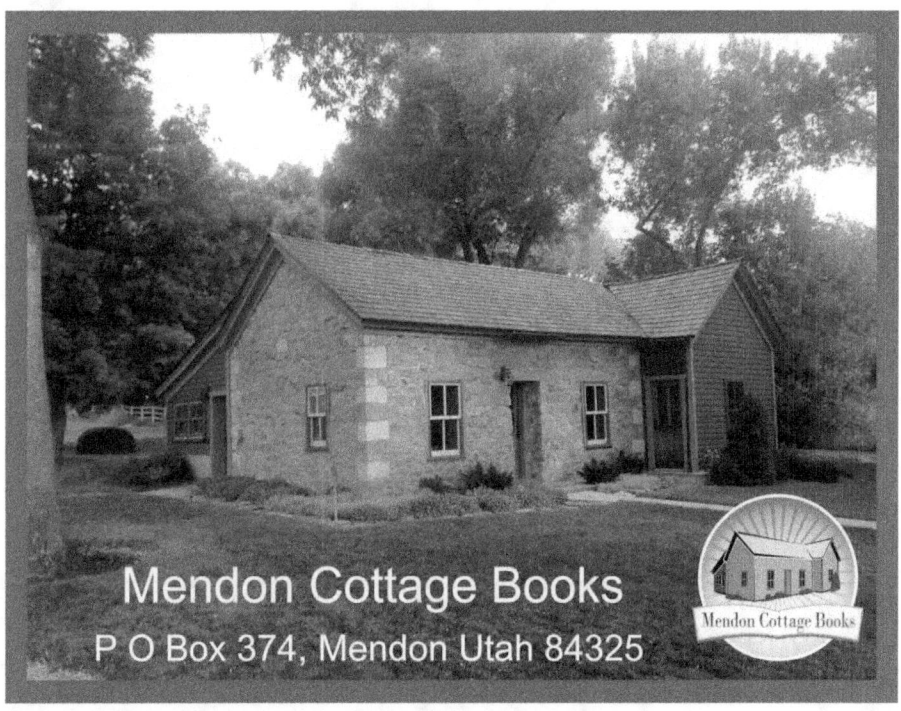

Mendon Cottage Books

P O Box 374, Mendon Utah 84325